Sex Explained!

How to Improve Couple Intimate Moments, Overcome Sexual Anxiety and Build Your Confidence, Learn the Hottest Foreplay Tips with the Best Sex Positions Available

Cheryl Bach

Sex Explained!

Cheryl Bach

Table of Contents

Sex Explained!

Chapter 1

Introduction

Sex is an important aspect of any romantic relationship. It allows couples to establish and maintain intimacy, express their desires and feelings, and share moments of pleasure. However, for many couples, sex can also be a source of anxiety, frustration, and conflict.

What Exactly Is Sex?

While the answer to this question may seem obvious, it's important to establish a clear and concise definition of sex before delving into its complexities. Simply put, sex is a physical act that involves mutual sexual stimulation between two consenting adults. This can take on a variety

Sex Explained!

of forms, ranging from kissing, touching, and oral sex to vaginal or anal penetration.

Why Is Sex So Important?

For starters, sex produces a variety of physical and emotional benefits that can deepen the connection between romantic partners. During sex, the brain releases endorphins, which are natural feel-good chemicals that create a sense of pleasure and relaxation. This can help couples to feel happier and more relaxed in their relationships, as well as increase overall intimacy.

In addition to its emotional and physical benefits, sex also plays a critical role in maintaining the health and longevity of a romantic relationship. Studies have shown that couples who engage in regular sexual activity report higher levels of satisfaction and commitment to their relationships than those who do not. By prioritizing sex and making an effort to maintain a healthy and satisfying sex life, couples can strengthen their relationships and improve their overall happiness and well-being.

However, it's important to note that not all couples may experience the same benefits from sex. Factors such as sexual orientation, individual preferences, and cultural backgrounds can all impact a couple's experience with sex and intimacy. Additionally, issues such as sexual anxiety, past trauma, or physical health problems can all negatively impact a couple's sex life and overall relationship satisfaction.

That is why it is important for couples to communicate openly and honestly about their sexual needs and desires. By having conversations about sex, couples can work together to identify potential issues or areas for improvement, establish boundaries and preferences, and explore new ways to connect with one another. Additionally, seeking out educational resources and professional guidance can also help couples overcome specific challenges and deepen their understanding of their sexual health and relationship dynamics.

In conclusion, sex is a critical component of any romantic relationship. Whether it takes on a physical or emotional form, sex has the power to deepen the bond between partners, enhance emotional and physical well-being, and improve overall relationship satisfaction. Through communication, education, and a commitment to improving their sex lives, couples can build stronger, healthier relationships and enjoy all the benefits that good sex has to offer.

In this book, we will explore various topics related to sex and intimacy, including how to overcome sexual anxiety, build confidence, and learn new foreplay tips and sex positions. By reading this book and applying the techniques outlined in its pages, you can take steps towards improving your sex life, enjoying more fulfilling intimate moments with your partner, and strengthening the bond between you both. So, let's dive in and begin our journey of understanding and experiencing the joys and pleasures of good sex!

Sex Explained!

Chapter 2

Overcoming Sexual Anxiety

Sexual anxiety can be a common issue for couples and individuals, especially in situations where they may feel vulnerable or uncertain about their sexual desires or abilities. In this chapter, we will explore the causes and symptoms of sexual anxiety, as well as strategies for managing and overcoming this challenge.

Causes and Symptoms of Sexual Anxiety

Sexual anxiety can have a variety of underlying causes, including past trauma, performance anxiety, relationship issues, body-image concerns, or negative beliefs and attitudes towards sex. These factors can lead to feelings of insecurity, shame, discomfort, or fear around sexual

Sex Explained!

activity, and can impact an individual's ability to fully engage in intimate moments with their partner.

Some common symptoms of sexual anxiety include:

- Difficulty achieving or maintaining an erection/ lubrication
- Pain during sex
- Lack of desire or interest in sexual activity
- Inability to reach orgasm
- Feelings of shame, guilt, or self-consciousness during sexual activity
- Avoidance of sexual activity or intimacy with one's partner
- Negative self-talk or increased levels of stress and anxiety

The impact of sexual anxiety can be significant on both individuals and their relationships. It can lead to increased stress, lowered self-esteem, decreased intimate connection with one's partner and decreased relationship satisfaction.

Cheryl Bach

Strategies for Managing Sexual Anxiety

There are a variety of strategies that individuals and couples can use to manage sexual anxiety and work towards building a healthy and enjoyable sex life.

Here are a few techniques that can be helpful:

Communication: Open and honest communication is a critical component of addressing sexual anxiety. By sharing your thoughts and concerns with your partner, you can work together to identify potential triggers, establish boundaries, and explore new ways to connect and express intimacy. Talking about your anxiety can help reduce the pressure during sexual activity, ultimately resulting in a more positive experience for both partners.

Education: Focused educational resources on sexual health, anatomy, and pleasure can be beneficial for individuals experiencing sexual anxiety. This knowledge will give individuals a better understanding of themselves and their partner's bodies and needs, leading to more informed decision-making during intimacy.

Mindfulness: Practicing mindfulness can help individuals identify and regulate negative thoughts and emotions that may arise during sexual activity. By focusing on breathing or other sensory experiences, mindfulness can also help individuals stay present in the moment and reduce distractions or performance anxiety.

Therapy: Seeking professional counseling or therapy services can be beneficial for individuals with severe sexual anxiety. Trained therapists can help individuals explore the factors contributing to their anxiety, develop coping strategies, and assist them in enhancing their intimate connections with their partners.

Sensate focus exercises: These activities are designed to improve sexual experiences by shifting the focus of attention from sexual performance to exploring one's body and sensations. This type of therapy helps couples rediscover a non-sexual form of touch that can gradually work its way up to sexual touch, helping them build trust and intimacy over time.

Gradual exposure: Gradual exposure is another effective therapy technique where individuals gradually expose themselves to the situations that cause them anxiety. In the context of sexual anxiety, this could involve gradually building up sexual activity with your partner over time, starting with less intimate moments and gradually moving towards more intense forms of sexual activity, which ultimately help in reducing anxiety over time.

In conclusion, sexual anxiety is a common issue affecting individuals and couples at various stages in their relationships. However, the good news is that it is a manageable condition that can be improved with the right techniques and tools. Finding ways to manage anxiety during sexual activity, engaging in open communication, seeking professional assistance, and learning new strategies to connect and communicate with a partner are all steps that can help individuals and couples tackle sexual anxiety.

By acknowledging its presence, identifying its causes, and developing an appropriate response, individuals can work towards overcoming sexual anxiety and improving their intimate life and the relationship. Remember, it is important to seek help if anxiety is becoming challenging to cope with or is having a negative impact on life or your relationship. With patience, effort, and communication, overcoming sexual anxiety can help individuals and couples discover deeper levels of intimacy and pleasure in their sexual experiences.

Chapter 3

Building Confidence in Your Sex Life

Sexual confidence can play a significant role in improving your intimate moments and overall relationship satisfaction. However, building sexual confidence can be challenging, especially for individuals who experience sexual anxiety. This chapter will explore the importance of communication in a sexual relationship, tips for improving scxual confidence, and strategies for increasing sexual trust with your partner.

Importance of Communication in a Sexual Relationship

Effective communication is essential in every aspect of a relationship, including sexual intimacy. A lack of communication about sex and desires can lead to confusion, misinterpretation, or unanswered needs, which can ultimately increase stress or dissatisfaction. Therefore, it is essential to have open conversations about your sexual needs with your partner.

In addition to conveying sexual needs, effective communication also involves active listening. When discussing sexual experiences, each person should focus on understanding their partner's perspective, needs, and desires. It is also important to communicate in a non-judgmental, compassionate and respectful way; this will create an environment that fosters trust and understanding.

Here are some tips for effective communication in a sexual relationship:

Schedule a time to talk: If you find it difficult to discuss your sexual desires spontaneously, try scheduling a dedicated time to speak with your partner about your needs in a non-interruptive setting.

Use "I" statements: Instead of blaming the other person or making demands, frame your concerns using "I" statements; this technique creates a safer space and less chance of someone becoming defensive.

Give feedback: During intimate moments, it is important to give feedback on what feels good and what does not. This help your partner adjust and improve their performance next time.

Show appreciation: Saying thank you to your partner after sexual activity promotes positive reinforcement. It can lead to increased intimacy, validation, and a feeling of closeness.

Be open-minded: Every person has their unique preferences and aversions in bed. Avoid being judgmental if your partner expresses a desire that you may not feel comfortable with. Instead, initiate an open conversation to better understand your partner's perspective.

Tips for Improving Sexual Confidence

Sexual confidence is not something that comes naturally to everyone in a relationship. Often it is something that takes time to build with your partner.

Below are some tried-and-true tips for upping your game in the bedroom:

Educate yourself: Learn all you can about your body, your partner's body, and sexual pleasure. Attend workshops, read books, or watch educational videos together.

Take care of yourself: Confidence starts with having a positive view of yourself. Taking care of your own well-being and appearance can boost confidence levels. Regular exercise, healthy eating habits, good hygiene, and dressing well can help you feel more confident.

Explore outside of the bedroom: Trying new experiences or hobbies as a couple can serve as reminders to each other that you are attractive and desirable.

Communicate with your partner: Share your needs and desires with your partner; listen to their feedback, and take it into consideration. Knowing that your partner understands what you want and need can greatly boost your confidence.

Practice self-affirmation: Create self-affirming statements that positively affirm and remind you of your worth and capability. Recite these statements to yourself regularly.

Sex Explained!

Strategies for Increasing Sexual Trust with Your Partner

Trust is key to any healthy relationship, including sexual ones.

Here are some strategies for increasing sexual trust with your partner:

Start small: Build trust by starting small and gradually increasing the level of intimacy over time. This can include holding hands, kissing, or engaging in other non-sexual acts of intimacy.

Be honest: Honesty is crucial in a sexual relationship. Be transparent about your needs, desires, and limits. This will create an environment of trust and understanding between you and your partner.

Show vulnerability: Vulnerability can connect two people emotionally. Share something that makes you feel sensitive or requires trust from your partner, as long you feel comfortable with sharing that information.

Experiment together: Trying new things together can be informative, such as trying new sex positions or having fun with sex toys. It conveys a willingness to explore each other's desires and can deepen intimacy to build sexual trust.

Collaborate: Collaborating during intimate moments can build trust between partners. Each person should take responsibility for their pleasure and the pleasure of their partner. Find out what works best for you as a couple and communicate constantly. Being willing to participate in activities that meet both partner's needs shows that you respect each other's desires.

Sex Explained!

In summation, sexual confidence is crucial to a happy and healthy relationship. Openly communicating, practicing self-affirmation, building vulnerability and slowly building intimacy will increase your confidence and set a foundation for sexual trust with your partner.

Chapter 4

Hottest Foreplay Tips

Foreplay is often ignored or rushed during sexual activities, but it plays a crucial role in building sexual tension, increasing arousal, and improving the overall experience. Irrespective of gender, age, or sexual orientation, everyone can benefit from engaging in fun and exciting foreplay techniques.

Importance of Foreplay

Foreplay is key to the process of sexual arousal for both men and women. It helps to build intimacy and emotional connection between partners. Engaging in foreplay also increases blood flow, which leads to heightened sensitivity and sexual desire. In addition, it can increase lubrication, making sexual intercourse more comfortable and enjoyable. By slowing down and spending time focusing on each other's bodies, partners can build sexual anticipation and achieve deeper levels of intimacy and pleasure.

Types of Foreplay

There are several types of foreplay activities that can be enjoyed by couples. Here are a few examples:

Kissing: Start with gentle kissing before gradually increasing the passion by using tongue and varying pressure.

Touching: Explore each other's bodies by touching areas that feel good while communicating what feels better.

Massage: Use scented oils or candles to heighten the senses, and incorporate massage as a method of foreplay.

Oral sex: Engage in oral sex on each other as part of foreplay to increase the level of arousal before moving on to intercourse.

Role-playing: Using role-playing techniques to act out fantasies or explore dominant/submissive scenarios can be particularly exciting for couples.

Tips for Engaging in Foreplay

Communicate your desires and boundaries upfront: Discuss with your partner what you are willing and not willing to do before engaging in any foreplay activity.

Take your time: Foreplay is not meant to be rushed, so take your time to explore each other's bodies.

Sex Explained!

Experiment with different types of foreplay: Each person has their own preferred type of foreplay that turns them on. Experimenting with different techniques will help partners find new ways to please each other.

Focus on the senses: Engage all the senses by incorporating scents, music, and texture during foreplay to heighten sexual arousal.

Be attentive: Pay attention to your partner's reactions and adjust your technique accordingly.

Don't forget the non-sexual intimacy: Hugging, cuddling, and simply enjoying each other's company can also build emotional intimacy and lead to more satisfying sexual experiences.

Try something new: Sometimes trying new things can help break the monotony and bring a new level of excitement to foreplay. Consider introducing new sex toys, lingerie, or even trying new locations for foreplay.

Don't be afraid to take the lead: Both partners can take turns leading during foreplay. This helps to build trust while keeping things interesting and exciting.

Be present in the moment: Be mindful and present in the moment while engaging in foreplay. This helps to build intimacy and emotional connection with your partner.

In conclusion, foreplay plays a crucial role in building sexual tension, increasing arousal, and improving the overall sexual experience. By communicating effectively, experimenting with different techniques, and focusing on the senses, couples can have more satisfying and pleasurable sexual experiences. Remember to take your time, be present in the moment, and enjoy the intimate moments shared with your partner.

Chapter 5

The Best Sex Positions Available

Sex is an essential part of any romantic relationship, and the secret to having great sex is variety. One of the best ways to add some spice to your sex life is by trying out different sex positions. In this chapter, we will be exploring some of the most popular and exciting sex positions available.

Different Sex Positions

Missionary position:

The most common sex position is the missionary position. This position is a classic because it allows for maximum eye contact and intimacy between partners. For best results, the partner on bottom should first place a pillow under their hips to create a better angle for penetration.

Doggy style:

Doggy style is another popular position. This one can provide deep penetration and is a great position for hitting the G-spot. To spice it up, the partner on bottom can add a vibrator or dildo for clitoral stimulation

Cowgirl:

Cowgirl is a great position for the partner on top to have control over the speed and depth of penetration. The receptive partner can also have their hands free for clitoral stimulation or to explore their own body. It's important to communicate with your partner about what feels good and what doesn't in this position.

Reverse cowgirl:

Giving a different twist to the cowgirl position, the receptive partner faces away from their partner in reverse cowgirl. This position provides deeper penetration and can stimulate the sensitive A-spot. Be sure to take things slow and communicate with your partner for the most enjoyable experience.

The spoon:

The spoon position is a cozy and intimate position where both partners lie on their sides facing the same direction, with the receptive partner's back pressed up against the penetrating partner's front. It's a great option for relaxing sex, and allows partners to whisper sweet nothings and be close to each other. For added stimulation, the receptive partner can raise their top leg for deeper penetration.

Standing sex:

Standing sex requires a little bit of effort and balance, but it's definitely worth it. This position can be done against a wall or a sturdy piece of furniture, with the penetrating partner lifting the receptive partner up for penetration. It's a

Sex Explained!

great position for adventurous couples who want to try something new.

Benefits of Different Sex Positions

Different sex positions can offer different benefits to couples, both in terms of physical and emotional satisfaction. For example, positions like missionary and spoon allow for maximum intimacy and closeness, while positions like cowgirl and doggy style provide deeper penetration and the ability to stimulate sensitive areas. Standing sex can add an element of spontaneity and adventure to your lovemaking.

It's important to remember that every couple is unique, and what works for one couple may not work for another. The key to finding the right sex position is to communicate with your partner and be open to trying new things. Don't be afraid to experiment and find what feels best for both of you.

Cheryl Bach

Proper Engagement in Different Sex Positions

One of the most important aspects of engaging in different sex positions is proper communication with your partner. Make sure you are both comfortable with the position before trying it out, and communicate throughout to ensure that you're both enjoying the experience. Proper lubrication is also essential for some positions to prevent discomfort or injury.

In terms of physical technique, take your time and start slowly to properly engage in each position. Experiment with angles and movement to find what feels best, and don't be afraid to switch things up if a position isn't working for you.

Overall, the key to properly engaging in different sex positions is to be present in the moment and focused on your partner. It's not just about achieving orgasm or trying to perform a certain way - it's about shared pleasure, intimacy, and love.

In conclusion, trying out different sex positions can add excitement and variety to your sex life as a couple. From traditional positions like missionary to more adventurous positions like standing sex, there are plenty of options to explore. With proper communication, technique, and focus on pleasure and intimacy, you can find what works best for you and your partner.

Chapter 6

Tips and Guidelines for Good Sexual Health

Sexual health is a vital component of overall health and wellbeing. It is not just the absence of disease or dysfunction, but a positive and respectful approach to sexuality and sexual relationships. In this chapter, we will explore what sexual health is, the importance of safe sex practices, and ways to improve your sexual health for a better sexual experience.

What Is Sexual Health?

Sexual health is a state of physical, emotional, mental, and social wellbeing related to sexuality and sexual behavior. It

Sex Explained!

includes the ability to have pleasurable and safe sexual experiences, free from coercion, discrimination, and violence. Sexual health also involves understanding and respecting oneself and others' sexual rights and needs, as well as practicing safe sex to prevent sexually transmitted infections (STIs) and unintended pregnancies.

The Importance of Safe Sex Practices

Safe sex practices are essential for maintaining good sexual health and preventing the spread of STIs.

Here are some tips to help you practice safe sex:

- Always use a barrier method, such as condoms or dental dams, during sexual contact.
- Get tested for STIs regularly, especially if you have multiple sexual partners. This will help you catch any infections early and prevent further spread.
- Avoid sharing sex toys or other intimate items with others, as this can increase the risk of infection.
- Discuss your sexual history and STI status with your partner before engaging in sexual activity.

- If you or your partner have an STI, seek treatment right away and avoid sexual contact until the infection is cleared.
- Use lubricant to reduce the risk of tears and other injuries during sexual activity.

Improving Sexual Health for Better Sexual Experience

Aside from practicing safe sex, there are several ways to improve your sexual health and have a better sexual experience overall. Here are some tips:

Communicate with your partner – Communication is key when it comes to having a healthy sexual relationship. Be open and honest with your partner about your desires, needs, and boundaries. This will help you both feel more comfortable and connected during sexual activity.

Practice self-care – Taking care of your body and mind can improve your sexual health and lead to better sexual experiences. This includes getting enough sleep, eating a healthy diet, exercising regularly, and reducing stress.

Explore your sexuality – Take time to explore your own sexuality and learn what feels good for you. This can include experimenting with different types of touch, trying new positions, or using sex toys.

Seek professional help – If you are experiencing sexual problems or difficulties, don't hesitate to seek professional help. Sexual problems can stem from a variety of factors, including physical or psychological issues. Seeing a healthcare provider or therapist who specializes in sexual health can help you identify and address any underlying issues.

Avoid substance abuse – Excessive alcohol or drug use can impair sexual functioning and lead to risky sexual behavior. Practice moderation and avoid using substances to enhance sexual experiences.

In conclusion, good sexual health is essential for a fulfilling and enjoyable sexual experience. Safe sex practices, communication, self-care, and exploration are all important components of sexual health. By taking care of your physical, emotional, and mental wellbeing, you can improve your sexual health and have a happier and more fulfilling sex life. Remember to prioritize your health and safety, and don't hesitate to seek help if needed.

Sex Explained!

Chapter 7

Conclusion

Throughout this book, we have explored various ways to improve and enhance your intimate moments as a couple. From overcoming sexual anxiety to learning hot foreplay tips and the best sex positions available, we hope that you have gained valuable insight and tools for building a healthier sexual relationship.

Recap of Key Points

To summarize the key points discussed in this book, we have learned about:

- The importance of communication, trust, and respect in a sexual relationship
- How to overcome sexual anxiety and build confidence

Sex Explained!

- Techniques and tips for foreplay and achieving climax
- Different sex positions to explore and experiment with
- The importance of safe sex practices and good sexual health

Encouragement for Couples to Explore and Experiment with Their Sexuality

We would like to encourage couples to continue exploring and experimenting with their sexuality, as it will help to deepen the bond between partners and create a more fulfilling sexual experience. Don't be afraid to try new things and step outside of your comfort zone. Remember, safe and consensual exploration of your sexuality can lead to a much stronger and satisfying relationship.

Cheryl Bach

Final Thoughts on the Importance of Good Sex in a Relationship

Good sex is a crucial component of a healthy and happy relationship. It allows couples to connect on a deeper level, increase intimacy, and build trust and respect. When both partners feel their desires and needs are being met in the bedroom, it can lead to a more positive and fulfilling overall relationship.

However, it's important to remember that every couple has their unique sexual preferences and needs. What works for one couple may not work for another. Communication, experimentation and open-mindedness are all key factors in creating a fulfilling and satisfying sexual relationship.

In conclusion, we hope that you have found this book to be a valuable resource in improving your intimate moments as a couple, overcoming sexual anxiety, and building your confidence. We encourage you to take what you have

Sex Explained!

learned here and incorporate it into your own relationship. Remember to communicate with your partner, be open to exploration, and prioritize each other's pleasure and satisfaction.

We believe that a healthy and fulfilling sexual relationship can contribute significantly to overall relationship satisfaction and happiness. So go ahead and use the tips and techniques described in this book to create more meaningful and satisfying intimate moments with your loved one.

Thank you for taking the time to read Sex Explained! We wish you all the best on your journey towards a happy sexual relationship.